Activities for the Family Caregiver

TRAUMATIC BRAIN INJURY

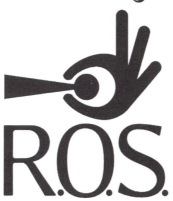

R.O.S.

HOW TO ENGAGE
HOW TO LIVE

Scott Silknitter,
Lisa Gonzalez, MS, OT/L, CCM, CBIS
Heather McKay, MS, OT/L

Disclaimer

This book is for informational purposes only and is not intended as medical advice, a diagnosis, or treatment. Always seek advice from a qualified physician about medical concerns, and do not disregard medical advice because of something you read in this book. This book does not replace the need for diagnostic evaluation, ongoing physician care, and professional assessment of treatments. Every effort has been made to make this book as complete and helpful as possible. It is important, however, for this book to be used as a resource and idea-generating guide and not as an ultimate source for a plan of care.

ISBN # 978-1-943285-13-6

Published by
R.O.S. Therapy Systems, L.L.C.
Greensboro, NC
888-352-9788
www.ROSTherapySystems.com

Introduction:

Activities for the Family Caregiver— Traumatic Brain Injury

Life happens. Your loved one did not plan on being in this position, and you did not plan on being a caregiver. But here you are.

Whether through an auto accident, sports injury, slip and fall, or military service, traumatic brain injuries (TBIs) occur for a variety of reasons. Each person's situation is as unique as that individual.

Our goal and mission is to help you with this change by providing basic, common sense suggestions and ideas that you can adapt to your loved one's specific situation to make things a little easier for yourself—and for your loved one.

This book provides a general guide for family caregivers— covering strategies and tips for planning and carrying out activities and personal care tasks for someone with a traumatic brain injury. It shares the principles and approaches that long-term care professionals learn and practice through their training and certification process. It does so by incorporating everyday common sense approaches and practical information for vital activities— like leisure and personal care routines. *Activities for the Family Caregiver—Traumatic Brain Injury* is part of the *R.O.S. Activities for the Family Caregiver* book series, which is designed to help caregivers more effectively engage those for whom they care.

With the assistance of industry-leading professionals, Lisa Gonzalez and Heather McKay (see biographical information in the About the Authors section), we have written this book to provide intentional and practical "How To's" for engaging with your loved one on a daily basis. Our company, R.O.S., began as a simple backyard project specifically to help my mother and father in a 25-year journey with Parkinson's and dementia. **It was my father's disease and my family's experience of various styles of caregiving that made this a personal journey and led to all the things that R.O.S. does to promote a better quality of life for caregivers and those they love. R.O.S. Therapy Systems and the R.O.S. Centers around the United States proudly serve family and professional caregivers with activity products, on-demand educational tools, and live classes designed to engage people in activities despite a life-changing diagnosis.** I hope you are able to benefit from my father's long fight by gleaning from our experiences and lessons outlined on the following pages.

Please also share this book and its principles with other family members and caregivers. Use it as a tool to break down the walls of isolation for you and your loved one. This resource can ensure that everyone who surrounds your loved one on a regular basis is on the same page.

From our family of caregivers to yours, please remember that *you are not alone.* No matter how hard the moments may be, there is hope for meaningful interactions—and an engaging life beyond traumatic brain injury. You have support from those who have paved the way before you. *Never give up.*

—Scott Silknitter, Founder of **R.O.S. Therapy Systems, L.L.C.**

Table of Contents

Chapter 1

Traumatic Brain Injury Overview

A Traumatic Brain Injury (TBI) happens when someone's head is severely hit or shaken, or when an object penetrates the brain and disrupts the normal functioning of the brain. In an uninjured brain, the different areas of the brain use connections (called axons) to communicate with one another. When a blow or jolt causes shearing or bruising of the brain, a loss of these connections often occurs. The microscopic damage to these connections can disrupt brain function. Each year, a reported 1.7 million individuals sustain a TBI in the US, according to the Centers for Disease Control (CDC).

Falls are the leading causes of TBIs (35–40 percent), primarily for those aged 0 to 14 and 65 and older. From 14–20 percent of TBIs are caused by motor vehicle accidents, while assaults and "struck by/against" situations contribute to another 26 percent of the TBI causes.

TBI is a leading cause of disability for young people—and particularly men. Of the 70 percent of TBIs involving young people between 16 to 24 years of age, two thirds will be male. For every severe TBI, there are 10 mild brain injuries. However, the word "mild" doesn't mean there aren't serious concerns that can affect the person with the injury, their friends, and their family.

The majority of TBIs occur in that prime productive stage of life where identities, roles, and often socialization center around the workplace. For that reason, there are often major changes and implications that involve a person's security, esteem, relatedness, and sense of purpose.

TBIs can range in severity from a mild concussion that may heal without medical treatment to severe injuries that require surgery and years of rehabilitation. While severe TBIs may be easy to detect, because a person's head is noticeably injured or the person is in a coma, mild concussions are often overlooked—and yet can have serious consequences.

Concussions are a serious problem, accounting for about 90 percent of TBIs and creating significant difficulties for the injured people and their families. Furthermore, problems from multiple brain injuries add up over time. People who suffered even a mild TBI are at risk for further brain trauma and will take longer to recover from future head injuries.

You may have heard about the risk of an injured football player heading back to the field before fully recovering from a concussion. The same applies with blast exposures and some military injuries. For example, many warriors who are nearby an explosion or who suffer a direct hit with minimal physical damage end up redeployed—only to suffer additional blast injury, which can compound the original damage.

Those with a concussion may look the same after the injury, walk and talk with no problem, and even report that they feel fine—when, in fact, they've suffered a TBI. Symptoms of a concussion—such as headache, dizziness, nausea, fatigue, and irritability—are symptoms that we've all had at some time in our lives, often unrelated to a brain injury. It's therefore easy to mistake those signs for something else or accidentally brush those complaints aside. Other symptoms can last for years—such as seizures, slurred speech, memory loss, lack of attention, and changes in vision or personality—and can get worse over time if left untreated. Often, these symptoms are subtle and might not affect functional abilities for several months.

Early Detection

It's important to diagnose and treat the person with a TBI as quickly as possible to improve long-term outcomes as well as decrease the risk of additional injuries.

Research in early detection and treatment is emerging to meet the growing needs of veterans who experience TBIs. According to a Rand study in 2008, one in five veterans of the wars in Iraq and Afghanistan has experienced a traumatic brain injury. The dramatic increase in TBI cases, up from previous wars, is attributed to more powerful munitions and improved body armor and protective gear. Service members are now surviving physical injuries that would have been fatal before today's protective equipment and specialized uniforms.

Thanks to the Brain Trauma Foundation, a nonprofit organization dedicated to improving the outcomes for people with TBI, in partnership with US Department of Defense and Veterans Affairs, early detection and treatment protocols are improving for all military and civilian patients. For example, Dr. Jamshid Ghajar, president and founder of Brain Trauma Foundation (BTF), has invented several neurosurgical devices that have been adopted worldwide—the latest of which is a simple test of a person's eye movements to detect brain injury.

In this test, patients are asked to watch a small dot of light as it moves in a predictable pattern, such as a circle, while their eye movements are monitored. Patients with normal brain function can predict the movement of the dot and are able to track the moving dot with ease. The task is much more difficult for patient with TBIs, so their eyes track in a wobbly pattern. The more severe the brain injury, the more the eyes appear wobbly, and the harder it is for the patient to pay attention. It is a 30-second test that can provide important information at the scene of an accident, at sporting events, or on the battlefield. Eye-tracking can be the first step in diagnosing TBI, followed by advanced imaging tools and additional professional assessments.

Supporting a Loved One with TBI

Once you know the symptoms of TBI, you or your loved one may be the first to recognize all or some of these changes. Here is a general list of symptoms, which we will explore more throughout this chapter:

1. Trouble with memory
2. Confusion
3. Poor judgment
4. Feelings of depression or anxiety
5. Trouble paying attention
6. Difficulty planning and completing daily activities
7. Changes in coordination and balance
8. Personality changes
9. Irritability
10. Easily frustrated
11. Trouble communicating or finding words, "spitting out" words

Each TBI affects each individual differently. For example, one person may feel out of control of his emotions or behavior, while another person does not have the emotional symptoms, but might have more problems with cognitive skills like attention and memory. Cognitive, physical, emotional, and social changes resulting from a TBI can then lead to changes in functional activities impacting habits and roles.

A TBI can ultimately change who we are as individuals—shaking our very personalities. On an ongoing basis, a TBI may also affect one's roles—such as employee, spouse, parent, and friend.

As the primary family caregiver, you need to know and understand the various symptoms of TBI so that you can adjust schedules, levels of participation, and time it takes to participate accordingly. You may also need to educate family, friends, and other caregivers about what your loved one may be experiencing and why. The following pages provide basic descriptions of TBI symptoms that may affect your loved one.

Primary Symptoms of TBI

Mild Traumatic Brain Injury

The signs and symptoms of mild TBI may include:

Physical Symptoms

- Loss of consciousness for a few seconds to a few minutes
- No loss of consciousness, but a state of being dazed, confused, or disoriented
- Headache
- Nausea or vomiting
- Fatigue or drowsiness
- Difficulty sleeping
- Sleeping more than usual
- Dizziness or loss of balance

Sensory Symptoms

- Sensory problems, such as blurred or double vision, ringing in the ears, a bad taste in the mouth, or changes in the ability to smell
- Sensitivity to light or sound

Cognitive or Mental Symptoms

- Memory or concentration problems
- Mood changes or mood swings
- Feeling depressed, anxious or irritable
- Slowed processing speed, difficulty keeping up with conversations
- Trouble communicating or finding words, "spitting out" words

<u>Moderate to Severe Traumatic Brain Injuries</u>

Moderate to severe TBIs can include any of the signs and symptoms of mild injury, as well as the following symptoms that may appear within the first hours to days after a head injury:

Physical Symptoms

- Loss of consciousness for several minutes to hours
- Persistent headache or headache that worsens
- Repeated vomiting or nausea
- Convulsions or seizures
- Dilation of one or both pupils of the eyes
- Clear fluids draining from the nose or ears
- Inability to awaken from sleep
- Weakness or numbness in fingers and toes
- Loss of coordination

Cognitive or Mental Symptoms

- Profound confusion
- Pre and post amnesia
- Decreased multitasking
- Concrete thinking, inflexibility
- Poor social skills
- Agitation, combativeness, or other unusual behavior
- Impaired communication

- Dysinhibition and impulsivity
- Slurred speech
- Coma and other disorders of consciousness

Children's Symptoms

Infants and young children with brain injuries may lack the communication skills to report headaches, sensory problems, confusion, and other symptoms. In a child with a TBI, you may observe:

- Change in eating or nursing habits
- Persistent crying and inability to be consoled
- Unusual or easy irritability
- Change in ability to pay attention
- Change in sleep habits
- Sad or depressed mood
- Loss of interest in favorite toys or activities

With applying specific activities based on personal preference and ability, many people with TBIs learn to live valued and productive lives. Just as individuals without TBIs grow and change, so do those with TBIs. The capacity to learn and improve different skills, even if only with small gains made, is still there years after an injury.

How You Fit In

As the primary family caregiver—often a spouse, partner, son, or daughter—your relationship and role with your loved one may change after the brain injury. You may become the cheerleader, motivator, protector, activity director, social coordinator, nurse, and even parent figure to your loved one. It is helpful to prepare yourself for these roles as much as possible, as they represent a big change not only for the injured—but for you.

How you provide support and assistance is key. Think about what it is like for your loved one to have everything that *was* done compared to how it *is* done now—versus how it *should be* done now. Everything your loved one does is being seen through glasses colored by the TBI. You, as the caregiver, will be challenged not to be the therapist all the time; sometimes you just need to be the spouse or loved one. We will keep these emotional aspects in mind as we explore practical steps you can take to ensure the most positive, productive outcomes in your interactions with your loved one.

Chapter 2

Activities, Their Benefits, and the Family

Whether it is at home, in a daycare program, or in a long-term care facility, "Activities" and personal care routines are critical aspects to supporting and caring for someone. This book is based on the training of long-term care professionals to help families and home care agencies caring for your loved one at home. It is designed to put everyone on the same page in regards to techniques, communication, planning, and execution of any activity that is attempted with your loved one. Both leisure and personal care activities require knowledge of your loved one's habits, preferences, abilities, and routines. **ALL** caregivers need to have the ability to communicate with and execute a planned activity with your loved one.

Activities, like all other things, can happen spontaneously; but they should be planned to offer the best possible outcome to enhance your loved one's sense of well-being. All caregivers—family, friends, or paid—should be on the same page. You are the captain of this ship, the quarterback, and the head cheerleader. What you know about your loved one's activity preferences will be helpful tips to the others supporting your loved one.

Activities should therefore promote or enhance your loved one's physical, cognitive, and emotional health.

In today's institutional settings, leisure activities are required by law, if a nursing home accepts government funding. In these situations, activities are to be provided to every resident on a daily basis according to an individual's preferences. Designing and implementing "Activities" has grown into a profession, wherein Certified Activity

Professionals and their staff plan and execute activity programs for residents in their care.

In addition, professional staff members are required to undergo annual training on the basics of Activities of Daily Living in order to provide better care for the residents they work with. There is therefore plenty of support for professional caregivers to engage people in activities in facilities, but it can be a challenge for caregivers to do the same, important work for loved ones in the home.

Given that there are millions of families and informal caregivers who care for their loved ones with TBIs at home, it's very important that some of the pertinent skills and training of formal, certified caregivers are made accessible. Recognizing the growth in the numbers of those caring for a loved one at home due to financial need or a simple desire to just be at home, the R.O.S. Activities 101/201 Programs and this book are based on the principles and approaches used by professionals to assist with the daily living activities of those with TBIs. This offers two benefits:

1. This provides family caregivers the knowledge and tools to allow them to engage their loved ones so that all can enjoy the benefits of activities.

2. It offers a starting point that will provide continuity of approach regarding care, communication, and information-gathering to minimize changes and acclimation time if your loved one does have to move from home to an institutional setting.

If you choose to use the services of a home care agency while caring for your loved one at home, please ask if they have a Home Care Certified professional on staff, and make sure that the caregiver you choose has received basic training on leisure activities and personal care routines. A CBIS (Certified Brain Injury Specialist) is someone with an additional level of specific training regarding TBIs and interacting with someone with a TBI.

The strategies and tools outlined in this chapter and book regarding activities will assist with continuity of approach, communication, and planning to benefit both you and your loved one.

Our goal is to help improve the quality of life for you and your loved ones. We do that by helping you deliver meaningful programs of interest to your loved one that focus on physical, social, spiritual, cognitive, and recreational activities.

Not all family members or friends may understand or accept your loved one's TBI. Your loved one may look the same on the outside and may be having a "good day" when someone comes to visit. People may underestimate or minimize the responsibilities or stress of being a caregiver. This can create conflict.

If it helps to avoid a conflict or stress, please have the family members read this book prior to a visit, so they can begin to understand the monumental task that you face as a caregiver. Use visits and interactions as teaching moments.

The Benefits of Activities with a Standard Approach

Caregiver Benefits of Standard Approach to Activities

Planned and well-executed activities result in less stress for the caregiver as well as less stress for your loved one. Whether the activity involves playing a game or bathing, a standard approach where as many details as possible are pre-planned can make a significant, positive difference for everyone. Knowing what to expect, to the best one can, helps empower all involved and enable a level of control when so much has changed.

Social Benefits of Activities

Activities offer the opportunity for increased social interaction between family members, friends, caregivers, and the one being cared for. Activities create positive experiences and memories for everyone. When possible, consider accessing community-based programs for additional support.

For example, there are thousands of disabled veterans participating in adaptive sports— with positive results, such as lower stress, reduced dependency on medications, fewer secondary diagnoses, higher achievement in work and school, and more independence (see www.va.gov/adaptivesports/va_groups_main. asp).

Behavioral Benefits of Activities

Well-planned and well-executed activities of any type can reduce challenging behaviors that sometimes arise when caring for someone with a brain injury. Additionally, frustration can decrease when an individual knows what to expect, with structure and routine.

Self-Esteem Benefits of Activities

Leisure activities offered with just the right level of challenge provide your loved one with an opportunity for success. This is also true with personal care routines such as dressing. Success during activities improves your loved one's sense of self-esteem.

Sleep Benefits of Activities

When regularly incorporated into a daily routine, activities can improve sleeping at night. If a loved one is inactive all day, it is likely that person will nap periodically. Napping can interrupt good sleep patterns at night.

Making the Outsider an Insider

Being a primary caregiver is a 24/7 job. Without help, you are always on call and run the risk of becoming physically and mentally exhausted. Taking care of yourself means you will be available to your injured loved one as well as other family members. Sometimes this means bringing in outside help.

When you do bring in help, make sure all of your loved one's caregivers (full-time, part-time, family, and friends) use the same approach for activities and interaction that you do. With a common approach, you significantly decrease the opportunities to disrupt routines and make unsettling changes that affect you and your loved one long after the help has left.

A common approach is a key to success!

The Four Pillars of Activities

The R.O.S. Activities 101/201 Programs focus on the Four Pillars of Activities. These are areas that all of your loved one's caregivers should be familiar with to provide continuity of care and the greatest opportunity for success—to engage and improve the quality of life for everyone.

First Pillar of Activities: Know your Loved One—Information Gathering and Assessment

- Have a Personal History Form completed.
- Know them—who they are, who they were, and what their functional abilities are today.
- Make sure all caregivers know this information as well.

Second Pillar of Activities: Communicating and Motivating for Success

- Communication is key. Each caregiver must know how to effectively communicate with your loved one and be consistent with techniques.

Third Pillar of Activities: Customary Routines and Preferences

- As best as possible, maintain a routine and daily plan based on your loved one's needs and preferences.

Fourth Pillar of Activities: Planning and Executing Activities

- Based on all of the information you have gathered about your loved one, you have the opportunity to offer engaging activities that are appropriate and meet your loved one's personal preferences.

Chapter 3

First Pillar of Activities: Know Your Loved One— Information Gathering and Assessment

Your loved one is a unique human being.

Before you begin providing personal care, you need to recognize various personal attributes and abilities of your loved one. The more you know about your loved one's lifestyle and likes/dislikes, the easier it will be to provide for his or her personal and leisure needs.

Knowing your loved one's individual needs, interests, functional abilities, and capacities will assist you in knowing how to plan and engage in meaningful and quality leisure activities. This is the First Pillar of Activities and will help in designing activities that your loved one can enjoy.

A TBI can have debilitating consequences.
Recovery is challenged by the fact that the
individual and the surrounding people know
"who" the individual used to be and "what"
that person could do prior to the TBI.
Individuals are constantly under scrutiny and
compared to premorbid (before TBI)
functional levels.

To be successful with an engagement, you
must concentrate on what your loved one
CAN DO—rather than what he or she can't do.
Here are some additional tips:

- Accentuate the positive, and set your
  loved one up for success.

- The more you know about your loved
  one, the more effective you can be
  as a caregiver.

- Caregiving routines should be kept
  structured and regular to the
  extent possible.

As the primary caregiver, you may already know most of the answers to the items listed next, but recording them in a Personal History Form (example following) is a good and necessary exercise to be completed by you, other family members, and other caregivers. Everyone has different memories and information about your loved one. When you put all of that information together, you paint a complete picture.

You might have heard offers from many people to help. The first thing they can do is share their memories of your loved one with you or fill out a Personal History Form as completely as possible.

At minimum, gather the information following as best as you can:

Basic Information

- Name, preferred name to be called, age, and date of birth

Background Information

- Place of birth, cultural/ethnic background, marital status, children (how many and their names), religion/church, military service/employment, education level, and primary language spoken

Medical and Dietary/Nutritional Information

- Any formal diagnosis, allergies, and food regimen/diets

Habits

- Drinking/alcohol, smoking, exercise, and other daily habits

Physical Status

- Abilities/limitations, visual aids, hearing deficits, speech, communication, hand dominance, and mobility/gait

Mental Status

- Alertness; cognitive abilities/limitations; orientation to family, time, place, person, routine; ability to follow directions; preference for written or verbal instructions; ability to comprehend and follow one-step versus multi-step directions; safety awareness; safety concerns; etc.

Social Status

- One-on-one interaction; communication with others through written words, phone calls, or other means such as email, Twitter, or Facebook

Emotional Status

- Level of contentment, outgoing/withdrawn, extroverted/introverted, dependent/independent, easily frustrated, easygoing

Leisure Status

- Past, present, and possible future interests

- Enjoys solitary versus social activities
- Physical versus passive (playing a sport versus watching a movie)

Details matter. Let's look at someone who enjoys woodworking.

During their assessments, four people might all say they like "woodworking," yet they might not actually have the same specific activity in mind—or even enjoy the same activity.

- Person 1—Enjoys sawing lumber, carrying and hauling the wood on the job site, using power tools, and working with a crew, nailing boards together to build structures. Anything less would not meet his preference. This person the physical construction and teamwork.

- Person 2—Enjoys working in the shop, sanding, gluing, and painting pieces of wood to construct smaller handmade projects such as a birdhouse, decorative bowl, chopping block, or writing pen. This person can spend hours seated at the workbench, repairing intricate details on old, wooden objects.

- Person 3—Enjoys the repetition of mass producing one woodworking project (wooden pens) for sale to support a local civic group. This person feels confident doing the same task with precision and accuracy and making many copies of the pen to raise money for the charitable group.

- Person 4—Enjoys the creative aspect of working with wood or repairing objects, problem solving, and "tinkering" towards fixing items—or creatively putting wood together from abstract ideas versus a detailed set of plans.

As you can see from these examples, *details matter.* Gather as much information as you can for yourself and all family members and caregivers who may help your loved one.

The R.O.S. Personal History Form (following) is a starting point to gather as much information as possible. You also may download a copy of the Personal History Form at www.ROSTherapySystems.com.

Personal History Form

This is _____'s Personal History

Name: _____

Maiden Name: _____

Date of Birth: _____

Preferred Name: _____

Name and relationship of people completing this history:

_____

_____

_____

Describe the person's personality prior to the onset of the injury. _____

_____

_____

What makes the person feel valued? Talents, occupation, accomplishments, family, etc. _____

_____

_____

What are some favorite items the person must always have in sight or close by? _____

_____

_____

What is his/her exact morning routine?

_____

_____

_____

_____

What is his/her exact evening routine?

_____

_____

_____

_____

What type of clothing does this person prefer? Does he/she like to choose his/her own clothes for the day, or is the preference to have clothes laid out by someone else?

_____

_____

_____

_____

What is his/her favorite beverage?

_____

What is his/her favorite food?

_____

_____

_____

What will get him/her motivated (church, friends coming over, going out, etc.)?

_____

_____

_____

_____

List significant interests such as hobbies, recreational activities, job related skills/experiences, military experience, etc.

      —Age 8 to 20:

      _____

      _____

      _____

      —Age 20 to 40:

      _____

      _____

      _____

What is this person's religious background? (Affiliation, prayer time, symbols, traditions, church/synagogue name, etc.) Did he/she lead any services or sing in the choir?

_____

_____

_____

What type of music does he/she enjoy listening to, playing, or singing? Does he/she have any musical talents?

_____

_____

_____

What is his/her favorite TV program? Movie?

_____

_____

_____

Did he/she enjoy reading? Which authors, topics, or genres does he/she prefer? Would he/she listen to audiobooks or books on tape?

_____

_____

_____

_____

Include names of spouses/partners, dates of marriage, and other relevant information. (If married more than once, provide specifics for each partner.)

_____

_____

_____

_____

_____

List distinct characteristics about his/her spouse/partner(s), such as occupations, personality traits, or daily routine.

_____

_____

_____

_____

_____

Does he/she have children? Be sure to include children both living and deceased. Include names, birth dates, and any other relevant information.

_____

_____

_____

_____

_____

Who does this person ask for the most? What is his/her relationship with this person(s)? Describe how that person typically spends the day.

_____

_____

_____

_____

_____

What causes your loved one stress? How is stress exhibited? Are there particular triggers like loud noises, white coats, or being ignored?

_____

_____

_____

_____

What calms him/her down when stressed or agitated?

_____

_____

_____

_____

How long has it been since the TBI? How did it happen?

_____

_____

Describe how the symptoms of the TBI are affecting your loved one.

_____

_____

_____

_____

_____

Has he/she accepted the changes in life since the TBI?

_____

_____

What activities does he/she feel can no longer be participated in as a result of the brain injury? And why?

_____

_____

_____

_____

What specific activities did he/she enjoy prior to the TBI diagnosis?

_____

_____

_____

_____

Is he/she participating less frequently with family and friends? Can you identify why?

_____

_____

_____

_____

Other information that would help to bring joy to your loved one.

_____

_____

_____

_____

_____

_____

_____

_____

_____

_____

_____

_____

_____

_____

_____

_____

_____

_____

_____

_____

Functional Levels

In addition to the information gathered in the Personal History Form—which tells everyone what your loved one enjoys, who that person is, and what his or her personal preferences might be—we also need to look at your loved one's functional level. This will allow you to plan activities that your loved one can accomplish. There are many functional scales available, but for our purpose, we will use the five levels as follow.

Level 1: Modified Independence

Your loved one is basically independent, using adaptive equipment or compensatory strategies. Social skills are adequate to make needs known and fit within the social norms. He or she initiates, plans, and even follows through with small projects/activities.

Those in this category have good social skills and are able to communicate. They are alert and oriented to person, place, and time, and they have a functional attention span for a concert or movie. They can initiate, plan, and even follow through with small projects/activities.

They also have problems with the big picture, responsibilities in family, follow through, attention to detail, and scheduling. They do not always think of the impact on others. They are ambulatory with or without a device. They may have lowered frustration tolerance and express frustration more readily.

Level 2: Supervision

Your loved one at this level still has pretty good physical skills, ambulates with or without a device, and may drive. No physical assistance is needed, just verbal support— possibly as reminders to do exercise or use a cane or walker.

Those at this level can be more egocentric, less aware of others. Decreased social skills exist such that those at Level 2 will yell at others who are slow or in the way. They need prompts to adjust tone or content of communication. They can participate in an activity with structure; set up and/or reminders; and prompting with sequencing, emotional regulation, and problem solving. They are somewhat rigid in ways and thinking.

Level 3: Minimal Assistance

At this level, your loved one may need both cognitive and physical assistance to complete tasks and participate in activities, but only about 25 percent of the time or with assistance for 25 percent of the task's effort. Support will need to be closer at hand in order to provide the assistance when needed. Memory and attention may be decreased, such that more routine prompting is needed in a 30 to 60 minute task; reminders are needed to finish or even stay on task. Support may be needed to give directions, such as to the bathroom in the movie theater or restaurant. Support might be needed in the form of a prompt to use a schedule and calendar.

Physical and sensory deficits may require mild hands-on support, for instance holding hands or escorting when walking on uneven terrain or cues for walking across a street. You might notice endurance and fatigue levels are lower. The ability to make needs known may be affected by speech deficits or cognitive deficits. Your loved one has fewer social skills. His or her verbal skills are even more impaired than they were at Level 2. He or she is also easily distracted. Your loved one may have some visual/spatial perception and balance concerns, and needs maximum assistance with care.

Level 4: Moderate–Maximum Assistance

At this level, someone is supporting your loved one in anywhere from 25–75 percent of a given task either cognitively, physically, or both. (The challenge may be physical or cognitive, but without the significant help from a caregiver, your loved one is unable to do the activity alone.)

Direct and more frequent prompts are needed for planning, problem solving, memory, and task attention. Initiation, safety awareness, and impulsivity can be a problem—requiring more supervision in the form of planning, encouragement, and safe execution of tasks. Physical and sensory deficits may be more severe, requiring assistance with self-care tasks as well as leisure activities. Increased physical assistance may be noted with the use of wheelchairs. Your loved one has a low energy level, few nonverbal communication skills, and rarely initiates contact with others; however, this person may respond if given time and cues.

Level 5: Total Assistance

At this level, the physical and sensory deficits are more severe and limit the functional level. If the individual requires total care or is needing support for more than 75 percent of the given task, he or she is considered to be at the "total assistance" level of care. While this is most easily demonstrated by physical disabilities, if your loved one is mobile but has balance problems or tremors, for instance, and cognitive deficits that require constant supervision, constant prompting to stay on task and/or to be safe, and hand-over-hand assistance to engage, this person would be considered at Level 5, total assistance.

Chapter 4

Second Pillar of Activities: Communicating and Motivating for Success

One of the biggest challenges for caregivers is the change in their roles and the system dynamics. A spouse is now a therapist, among other roles, for example. And that same spouse is also the gatekeeper and can often be perceived as the "one in charge"—reinforcing compensatory strategies, encouraging and prompting exercise programs and techniques, and determining if an activity is safe or not. It is a significantly difficult balancing act for the caregiver, as well as for the individual with a TBI. Add to the fact that this is often a 24/7 balancing act, and one can see how important and challenging communication can be.

Communicating is vital to your success in engaging in an activity with your loved one. Good communication is the Second Pillar of Activities.

The key to effective communication is listening attentively and using communication techniques that provide an open, nonthreatening environment for your loved one. Verbal as well as nonverbal communication will play a role in your ability to successfully engage your loved one. How you listen and try to communicate can either enhance and encourage communication or shut down communication altogether.

You need to assess your listening and communication style objectively and be able to assess the styles of other caregivers and family members working with your loved one. If communication was not a strength in the relationship prior to the TBI, outside support may be helpful in the form of counseling.

Verbal Communication

Communication is simply an interactive process whereby information is exchanged. More importantly, though, communication is a way to connect with another person. How well you connect depends on your ability to respond appropriately and give feedback on something that was communicated. It also depends on your ability to *listen*.

Verbal Approaches for Good Communication

- Use exact, short, positive phrases. Repeat twice if necessary. Have the individual repeat back what was said.

- Allow time for the person to answer. Avoid finishing others' sentences.

- Give one instruction at a time. Provide only the number of steps an individual can handle at a time.

- Use a friendly, respectful tone of voice.

- If the individual has a visual impairment, be sure to use verbal cues to let him or her know you are engaged.

- Talk to the person like an adult.

Verbal Communication Tips

- Speak directly to your loved one.

- When giving directions, make them as clear as possible.

- When speaking with other caregivers or family members about your loved one while he/she is present, make sure the conversation is respectful of your loved one, and be sure to include the loved one in the conversation to avoid it being "about" that person.

- Provide a written summary of information/instructions as needed if memory is an issue.

- When asking questions, adjust choices to what an individual can tolerate—open ended questions, versus multiple choice, or yes/no.

- Avoid battles or direct confrontations. For example, avoid situations wherein you are telling someone to do something. Providing choices will help.

Nonverbal Communication

Although it may seem that most communication happens verbally, research has shown that actually most communication occurs nonverbally. Facial expressions, eye contact, gestures, and even the amount of physical space between you and your loved one are nonverbal ways to communicate. Nonverbal communication can go a long way to convey your message and make your connection stronger, but it can also undercut your attempts to communicate if your nonverbal cues contradict your intention or send mixed signals. Even if your loved one is experiencing vision loss due to the TBI, your efforts to communicate positively through nonverbal cues and signals do matter.

Remember, too, that the effects of a TBI can make it difficult for your loved one to communicate feelings or a reaction to something you are trying to convey.

The key elements to consider regarding how you communicate nonverbally include:

Facial Expressions

- Be aware of what your facial expressions are conveying to your loved one. Your mood will be mirrored.

- Be careful if you're tired or stressed that your face doesn't show a bad mood. If your loved one asks, "What's wrong?" he or she may be reading a tense look on your face. Taking a few deep breaths can help you relax your facial expression.

Eye Contact

- Ensure that you have made eye contact with your loved one and that his or her attention is focused on you and what you are saying.

- It might be difficult for your loved one to understand what you're saying without seeing your face and eyes.

Gestures and Touch

- Calmly use nonverbal signs such as pointing, waving, and other hand gestures in combination with what you are saying.

- After a brain injury, your loved one may have trouble understanding the words heard. If your loved one misunderstands some of the words, visual cues and gestures can help this person keep up with the conversation or understand what you'd like done.

Tone of Voice

- The inflection in your voice helps your loved one relate to the words you are saying.

- Words convey facts, but the *feeling* in every interaction is in the tone. You know the difference in a friendly, respectful response and a frustrated or rushed answer. The difference is often not in *what* someone says, but rather *how* it is said. Keeping your tone calm, friendly, and respectful—the way we talk to adults—can help your loved one feel better about your communication.

For example, when asking what another person might want to do, many individuals ask in a bored or tone, "Do you want to go to the movie?" Now hear the difference when the question is asked with energy and enthusiasm in one's voice: "Hey, I thought you might want to go to the movies this afternoon, *IRobot* is playing—a new sci-fi."

Body Language

- Be aware of the position of your hands and arms when talking to your loved one.

- Similar to the tone of your voice, your body language sends a message, usually about your mood or feelings. For example, if your arms are crossed, it might send the message that you're upset or closed to an idea. If your head is propped in your hands, it might look like you're tired or bored. Pay attention to your loved one's body language too. You may be able to see a change in mood by watching body language. Adjust your support to make him or her more comfortable.

General Nonverbal Communication Tips

- Always approach your loved one from the front before addressing. This is especially true for veterans with PTSD on top of their TBIs—or with individuals who startle easily.

- Place yourself at eye level with the person to whom you are talking.

- Don't touch unexpectedly; it might startle your loved one.

- Give nonverbal praises such as smiles and head nods.

- Be an active listener.

Additional Approaches to Successful Communication and Activities

Be Calm

- Before you approach your loved one, consider how you're feeling. You may need to take a few deep breaths to settle yourself before you can support your loved one. Once you're feeling in control of yourself, approach your loved one in a relaxed and calm demeanor. Remember, your mood will be mirrored by your loved one. Smiles are contagious.

Be Flexible

- There is no right or wrong way of completing a task. Offer praise and encouragement for the effort your loved one puts into a task. If you see your loved one becoming overwhelmed or frustrated, stop the task, and re-approach at another time. Likewise, if you feel yourself getting overwhelmed or frustrated, take a time out, take some deep breaths, and approach it again when you're feeling in control.

- Sometimes, the best medicine is laughter. You and your loved one are a team, so if something isn't working, you might lower the stress by finding something to laugh about. With a positive attitude, you can try again.

Be Nonresistive

- Don't force tasks on your loved one. Adults do not want to be told, "No!" or directed on what to do. The power of suggestion goes a long way, and you get more with an ounce of sugar than a pound of vinegar.

Be Guiding, but Not Controlling

- Always use a friendly, respectful approach, and remember your tone of voice. Your facial expressions must match the words you are saying. If something's not working, back off, change something about your communication, the task or the environment and try again.

Barriers to Good Communication

There are generally two barriers that negatively affect communication with your loved one. Here are some tips on how to eliminate negative barriers.

<u>Caregiver Barriers</u>

- Slow down when speaking, if the person you are caring for has processing delays. Use a calm tone of voice, but not a childish tone, and be aware of your hand movements.

- Never be demanding or commanding.

- Never argue with a person with impaired cognition. You will never win the argument.

Environmental Barriers

<u>For those with attention and focus deficits and/or hearing problems:</u>

- Minimize noise from air conditioners and home appliances.

- Turn off the TV, if it is on in the same room where you are trying to talk.

- Be aware of outside traffic noise.

- Check your loved one's hearing aid battery, and make sure that it is not whistling.

Communication and Behavior

Behaviors are a means to communicate when words are no longer effective. When someone has difficulty or is unable to speak, the easiest way to communicate and express feelings, whether they are positive or negative, is through behavior. It might help to think of a bright young toddler who has a limited vocabulary, and so he expresses his wants and needs through what might be either good or bad behavior. For someone with a brain injury, it can become just as difficult for an adult to communicate wants and needs. Caregivers must uncover the meaning behind the behaviors and put a plan into effect to manage those needs. Be a detective.

Aggressive Behaviors

Aggressive behaviors can include hitting, angry outbursts, obscenities, yelling, racial insults, making inappropriate sexual comments, and/or biting. Trying to communicate with or provide care to a person who is aggressive can be stressful and even frightening for caregivers.

The following are some of the personal and environmental factors that may lead your loved one to show aggressive behavior.

- Too much noise or overstimulation
- Cluttered environment
- Uncomfortable room temperatures

- Basic needs not being met: hunger, thirst, needing to use the bathroom, needing comfort

- Pain

- Fear, anxiety, or confusion

- Communication barriers

- Fear or anxiety from not recognizing the surroundings

- Caregiver's mood

- Feeling that he or she is being rushed

- Difficulty seeing activity or materials of activity, which prevents him or her from participating

- Lack of independence

Interventions to Mitigate Aggressive Behaviors

- Communicate for success.

- Validate and support feelings.

- Remain calm, and speak in a friendly tone; avoid belittling or using a childish tone.

- Provide consistent caregivers and schedules. Stick to your loved one's routine.

- Engage in recreational activities that match the person's abilities and interests, as tolerated. Know that some tasks will require more support than other activities. Something familiar may require less assistance than something unfamiliar.

- Break down instructions into one-step increments.

- Identify the triggers of the aggression. Be a detective. There is never a behavior that *just occurs*.

- Keep an ongoing dialogue between family members and caregivers over any noted changes in patterns or behaviors.

- Help your loved one to slow down and relax.

As we've covered already, it's imperative that you know your loved one. Know what sets your loved one off. What are his or her emotional triggers? Is it the way someone talks? Or the staff? Is it that he or she doesn't like a particular person? You won't be able to eliminate everything that upsets your loved one, but knowing what triggers negative behaviors does allow you to avoid those triggers to a large extent. REMEMBER: negative behaviors are a form of communication. What is your loved one trying to communicate with this behavior?

When a loved one is acting out, remove the trigger, or remove him or her, in an attempt to deescalate the situation. When upset, communication will be challenging. Safety is key for all involved, when a loved one is upset. If an activity or communication is not working, back off, give yourself and your loved one some time to settle down, and try again.

Chapter 5

Third Pillar of Activities:
Customary Routines and Preferences

Maintaining your loved one's customary routines, and basing activities on your loved one's preferences, is the Third Pillar of Activities. Engaging your loved one in activities that promote a sense of accomplishment, provide opportunities for communicating and sharing, and help to maintain and improve functional and cognitive abilities can and should be part of each day's routine.

For example, you may ask your loved one to help you prepare a meal. Even if your loved one isn't used to cooking, that person may appreciate feeling helpful. We all need to be needed. If there are parts of the job that your loved one can do—such as retrieving something from the refrigerator, pouring the drinks, or setting the table—allow him or her to do so. And don't forget to say "thank you" for the teamwork.

The question should not be, "When should I do activities?" The focus should be on capitalizing on your loved one's abilities to create opportunities for a sense of meaning and acknowledging his or her continued role and importance as part of this family system.

In helping you to develop a daily plan of care for your loved one, we will be discussing two areas: Daily Customary Routine and Activity Preferences. The goal is to gain, from your loved one's perspective, how important certain aspects of care/activity are to that individual.

Daily Customary Routine

Your loved one has distinct lifestyle preferences and routines that should be preserved to the greatest extent possible. All reasonable accommodation should be made to maintain your loved one's lifestyle preferences, honoring and respecting who this person was prior to the injury, as well as recognizing there may be different preferences post injury.

Perhaps for years prior to the TBI, your loved one woke up every day and went to work at a construction company before the sun was up. His morning routine was minimal: a quick bowl of cereal and a cup of coffee. He took his coffee with milk and two teaspoons of sugar, sat at the head of the table for the simple meal, and enjoyed the quiet solitude of the morning routine. You should try to find ways to keep those activities a part of your loved one's routine. If he can no longer construct the morning routine on his own, what could you or other caregivers do to help him maintain the morning routine as much as possible?

If your loved one no longer goes to the same job, what are some productive activities you might do together after breakfast? Maybe household chores or tasks are set up towards a work-like setting. Volunteering can replace paid work, providing that same sense of purpose and "place to be."

Your loved one's ability to do many things independently—abilities that were taken for granted before the brain injury—might become diminished or lost due to the effects of the brain injury. With your help, however, allowing your loved one to preserve as much routine as possible will go a long way to improving and maintaining confidence, mood, and overall well-being.

Not accommodating your loved one's lifestyle preferences and routine can contribute to a depressed mood and increased behavior issues. When a person feels like all control has been removed and preferences are being disregarded and not respected, it can be demoralizing. This can especially be challenging for the caregiver whose loved one has experienced damage in the front part of the brain, where impulsivity and safety awareness have been impaired.

Prior to the injury, your loved one could control emotions and explain hurt feelings and possible solutions when upset. Like pulling on the reins of a horse, we hold our emotions in control for better problem solving. Since the injury, he or she might explode in a dangerous angry outburst, like the reins have been cut, because the emotional impulse control is damaged.

Activity Preferences

Activities are a way for individuals to establish meaning in their lives. The need for enjoyable and purposeful activities does not lessen or change based on age or health needs. However, we can modify the activities and the level of assistance one might need to engage in those pursuits.

A lack of opportunity to engage in meaningful and enjoyable activities can result in boredom, depression, and behavioral disturbances. For the safety and well-being of the person with a TBI and his or her family, a healthy engagement in activities is crucial.

Individuals vary in the activities they prefer, reflecting unique personalities, past interests, perceived environmental constraints, religious and cultural backgrounds, and changing physical and mental abilities. We as family caregivers have a great opportunity to empower a loved one to see that they still possess many great talents and abilities. By modifying or adapting an activity to allow someone to engage at an independent level, you are restoring self-esteem and self-worth.

Chapter 6

Fourth Pillar of Activities: Planning and Executing Activities

Planning and executing activities is the Fourth Pillar of Activities. Activities occur all day, every day. While certainly some activities can be spontaneous, most people find that the best activities are planned ahead. Spending some time to plan activities helps to ensure that they are appropriate for your loved one and offer the greatest opportunity for success. Please note again that schedules, routines, and plans should be followed. However, they may need to be adapted due to specific symptoms your loved one may be experiencing on a particular day.

As you plan your loved one's activities as part of their customary routine, you need to consider how an activity fits within the following criteria:

- Person Appropriate—Desires and Preferences
- Person Appropriate—Abilities and Functional Levels

Person Appropriate— Desires and Preferences

Person appropriate refers to the idea that each person has a personal identity and history. Everyone has unique desires and preferences, and a "person appropriate" activity is one that is designed with an individual's preferences in mind. It also means that the primary caregiver has to make sure that all caregivers understand the elements and purpose of each specific activity. Lesson plans are invaluable tools to communicate clearly and consistently to all caregivers the elements of an activity.

Remember our woodworking example? Four people said that they enjoyed "woodworking," but to each of them, "woodworking" meant something different. The example helps to illustrate how important it is when planning activities that you ensure that the activity is person appropriate and is based on the specific desires and preferences of your loved one.

Person Appropriate— Abilities and Functional Levels

This concept is also based on the idea that each person has a personal identity and history, but it also takes into account the varying functional levels at which a person may be able to participate in an activity. Physical, cognitive, and emotional changes from a TBI may require modifications or adaptations—or even supervision and assistance to perform a task. Based on your loved one's functional level and abilities, some activities may also be done as a group. This creates an opportunity for socialization, interaction, and conversation between you and your loved one. Remember our woodworking example when looking at personal preferences? What is it about an activity that interests your loved one? If it is the socializing, with woodworking perhaps an alternate activity with the same socialization aspect will meet the need.

Let's use the woodworking example again to look at "person appropriate" tasks based on abilities.

- Person 1—Enjoys sawing lumber, carrying and hauling the wood on the job site, and working with a crew, nailing boards together to build structures. Anything less would not meet his preference.

  Since his brain injury, person 1 is no longer able to perform the sawing using an electric saw, but may be able to use a manual saw, or assist or offer advice to someone doing that task. If managing the whole job is more difficult now, person 1 may still participate with the crew, but focus on only one part of the job.

Analyzing the various activities and tasks, and identifying which ones might be adapted or modified, will be key in providing a level of "just right" participation. In this case, the outdoor activity can be discussed, planned, and executed together.

- Person 2—Enjoys working in the shop; sanding; gluing; and painting pieces of wood to construct smaller handmade projects such as a birdhouse, decorative bowl, chopping block, or writing pen. This person can spend hours seated at the workbench, repairing intricate details on old wooden objects.

Since this person's injury, person 2 finds that she is no longer able to concentrate at the workbench for long periods. An adaptive setup with proper lighting, an uncluttered tabletop, and a step-by-step setup of the activity might make it easier for her to concentrate for brief periods.

Breaking the activity into smaller steps would help her accomplish short-term goals on the project, and a checklist posted at the workspace could make it easier for her to track her progress and finish with more time.

- Person 3—Enjoys the repetition of mass producing one woodworking project (wooden pens) for sale to support a local civic group. This person feels confident doing the same task with precision and accuracy and making many copies of the pen to raise money for the charitable group.

  Person 3 can no longer sequence the steps of the activity to assemble the fundraiser, but still wants to support the mission of his favorite charity. In this case, an assembly line can be set up to allow person 3 to do only one step of the task, such as sanding. A caregiver can offer the wood assembled and ready for sanding. With the simple motion and no time limit, person 3 can still contribute to the project he values.

- Person 4—Enjoys the creative aspect of working with wood or repairing objects, problem solving, and "tinkering" towards fixing items—or creatively putting wood together from abstract ideas versus a detailed set of plans.

  Person 4 can no longer initiate abstract ideas for creating new projects. Or this person physically cannot manage the ideas for projects. Maybe pairing up with another woodworker to assist with the creating would work. Maybe the other woodworker can help include your loved one's work into a collaboratively creative project. How might you infuse any creativity into woodworking? Maybe exploring different mediums will enable new creativity.

The Lesson Plan

A *lesson plan* is a tool that you can use to help plan activities. A good lesson plan consists of a list of items needed to complete the activity, clear instructions, and room to record any and all observations regarding your loved one's participation and engagement. All caregivers should use the lesson plan to stay up-to-date and informed as to your loved one's ability to participate in an activity. Over time, your loved one's interest or ability to engage in a particular activity may change, so we suggest using the activity lesson plan to document everything you or any other caregiver observes each time you engage with your loved one.

As your loved one's abilities and responses change, those changes will dictate how you modify an activity to meet his or her current needs and abilities. The lesson plan is an ever-changing document. It is meant to be written on to note the changes you made to the original plan, so that the family member or caregiver working with your loved one next can follow your modifications in the hopes of recreating a positive experience.

Items in the Lesson Plan

Date

Document the date the program is used with your loved one.

Program Name

You can rename the program if you or your loved one prefer.

Objective of Activity

Our goal is to provide meaningful activities. People have a need to be productive, and they want to engage in something with a purpose. List the objectives of the program.

Materials

List suggested materials to use with this program.

Prerequisite Skills

Detail the skills your loved one needs to participate in this program.

Activity Outline

Include step-by-step instructions to complete this program.

When you or a family member are conducting an activity with your loved one, documenting results and responses is critical to identifying ways to improve activity programs for your loved one. Items to document should include:

- <u>Verbal cues, physical assistance, or modifications you required for this activity.</u> What strategies seemed to work best? Which ones did not work so well?

- <u>How your loved one responded to this program.</u> Did this increase frustration levels or seem to calm the individual?

- <u>Whether your loved one enjoyed this activity.</u> What did he or she like or dislike about the activity?

- <u>Pay attention to other factors that might have affected the outcome</u>—distractions like phone calls, time of day, weather, tardiness of staff, etc.

A blank template is included on the next page to give you an example of what a lesson plan looks like.

*Note: Make sure caregivers and family members are consistent with the type of verbal cues, physical assistance, or modifications that produce positive results.

Lesson Plan Blank Example

Date	Program Name

Objective of Activity

Materials

Prerequisite Skills

Room Lighting

Activity Outline

Evaluation

Chapter 7

Leisure Activity
Categories, Tips, and Suggestions

Activity Categories

There are as many different possibilities for activities as there are individuals for whom to create them. To keep things simple, we place activities into three general categories: Maintenance Activities, Supportive Activities, and Empowering Activities.

Maintenance Activities

Maintenance activities are traditional activities that help a person to maintain physical, cognitive, social, spiritual, and emotional health. These are tasks and activities that reinforce and rehearse specific skill areas.

Examples include: using manipulative games such as those in the R.O.S. Legacy System, craft and art activities, working trivia and crossword puzzles like the *How Much Do You Know About* puzzles, taking a walk, and engaging in tai chi, yoga, exercise, therapy home programs, and kayaking.

Supportive Activities

If your loved one has a lower tolerance or capability for traditional activities, supportive activities provide a comfortable environment while providing stimulation or solace.

Examples include: listening to and singing music and engaging in music therapy, hand massages or massages in general, relaxation activities such as aromatherapy, meditation, and bird-watching.

Empowering Activities

Empowering activities help your loved one build and maintain self-respect by offering opportunities for self-expression and exercising responsibility.

Examples include: involvement in household activities like cooking, paying a bill, washing the car, and folding laundry. Volunteering can also be meaningful, and may include–helping with Meals on Wheels, going to an animal shelter, helping out in a child's class, or engaging in other volunteer programs. Other empowering activities may include taking classes for pleasure and/or credit, such as a continuing education cooking or a gardening class through a local community college. Assisting as a coach for a child's soccer team can also provide meaning and empowerment.

General Activity Tips

It is likely that your loved one will need some level of assistance from you when engaging in activities—be it cognitive, physical, or emotional support. Since one of the key goals of doing activities is to foster a sense of accomplishment and independence, we offer the following tips to help you anticipate some of the things that might come up in the course of engaging your loved one, to increase your loved one's chances for success, and to help make the experience a positive one for both of you.

Travel Tips for Moving from Room to Room or Place to Place

- When escorting your loved one, ask if assistance is needed. If no assistance is requested, walk side by side or a half step behind in case balance is lost.

- If your loved one does require some assistance, offer your arm to be held or interlock arms. Find the easiest and most comfortable way to walk together. Walk side by side or a half pace ahead while providing verbal cues about the environment.

- If your loved one requires equipment to move around, work with the medical professionals to get the best fit and function with mobility devices.

- Avoid puddles, snow banks, and other natural barriers.

- Avoid cracked tile, untacked throw rugs, and protruding floorboards.

Writing and Drawing Activity Tips

- If your loved one has trouble holding a pen or pencil, there is a wide variety of inexpensive grip holders available at local medical supply stores and therapy catalogues. A basic home remedy might be to wrap foam or Coband around the shaft of the pen to help your loved one's grip. (Coband is an elastic, sticky ace wrap found in pharmacies. It sticks to itself, providing a somewhat moldable way to improve one's grasp of a pen or pencil.)

- Instead of writing, typing on the computer or using an adaptive keyboard may be the way to write thoughts. There are all kinds of apps to help—from adaptive keyboards, speech to text, and keyboard guards—depending on the physical challenges your loved one may have.

- Reduce glare and shadowing by positioning a chair and table so any natural light is from behind instead of coming from the front.

- To prevent shadows, place lamps on the opposite side of the hand being used. Locate the bottom edge of the lampshade just below eye level.

- Shiny paper can increase glare, so it is best to use matte paper when reading or writing.

- Use large-print crossword, word search, or word scramble puzzles. See the R.O.S. *How Much Do You Know About* series of e-Books.

- A dry-erase board or tablet may also be used to practice writing.

*Note: Know the type of seating where your loved one is the most comfortable when writing, and if possible, move him or her to that seat.

*Note: If your loved one is seated in a wheelchair, recliner, or bed, provide a flat surface that fits in the lap, upon which to place paper.

Reading Activity Tips

- If reading is troublesome, try large-print books, available at most bookstores and libraries.

- Read to your loved one, or take turns reading to each other.

- Listen to audio tapes and books on CD borrowed from your local library, or from the free Talking Books program sponsored by the National Library Service. Many of the e-readers also offer audio support to books.

- If your loved one prefers reading to listening, many new mobile devices such as iPads, Kindles and Nooks all have options to increase the font size and adjust the color contrast.

- Try the Book Strap from the R.O.S. Legacy System to help keep a book and the page in place.

Hobby Activity Tips

- Make sure that supplies are easily accessible.

- Empower your loved one by choosing an area of the home where he or she can most comfortably participate.

  ○ If at a table and in a wheelchair, make sure the wheelchair can fit under the table.

  ○ If in a recliner, use an activity surface that fits comfortably in your loved one's lap, and choose an activity that does not have too many pieces that may be hard to keep track of.

- Craft Boxes and Materials

  - Place craft activity supplies in boxes clearly labeled with a broad-tipped black marker.

  - Group like items for activities together.

  - Store materials in different shaped/sized containers.

  - Choose identifying and organizational systems that work best for your loved one.

These strategies are especially helpful when working with individuals who have home health aides or other caregivers working with them. Having projects and supplies clearly identified and accessible makes them more likely to be used.

Game Playing Activity Tips

Playing Cards:

- If needed, use adaptive equipment such as card holders in which to place the playing cards while your loved one is seated at a table.

- The Card Holder Board Insert from the R.O.S. Legacy System allows your loved one to have the card holder in a lap while seated in a recliner or wheelchair.

Puzzles:

- Depending on the individual's fine motor or visual skills, select puzzle piece size and complexity to match ability and decrease frustration. Larger pieces and simple pictures may bring more success.

- If your loved one becomes frustrated because puzzle pieces are sliding when being placed, try a magnetic puzzle and a metallic flat surface so the pieces stay in place.

Adaptive Sports

There is a wide variety of organizations providing adaptive sports opportunities, from wheelchair basketball and rock climbing to surfing and scuba diving. Go online to find local organizations. Your state and local TBI association will also have valuable resources and support groups.

Active Activity Suggestions

Active activities, such as walking, dancing, stretching, biking, horseback riding, and playing sports are those that involve using large muscle groups. Physical activity is important, especially where physical limitations persist. Individuals in wheelchairs and those using a walker or cane burn fewer calories and have less overall movement patterns, making them prone to weight gain, decreased strength, lower endurance, and depression. Excessive weight gain from lack of activity makes transfers, self-care, and even mobility more challenging—as well as potentially having an impact on other health areas. In addition to the tips we offer for general activities, following are some suggestions for active activities. As you build these activities into your loved one's schedule, please be sure to leave opportunities for rest after or between activities. Depending on the activity or exercise, you, a family member, or a trained professional should always be there to supervise and assist your loved one as needed.

Generally speaking, there are four types of *active activities*: aerobic, strengthening, flexibility, and balance. Any of them can help to improve the quality of life for your loved one.

For health and wellness activities, if your loved one is comfortable, consider a local gym or recreational center to optimize community support and socialization. Look for a facility that will accommodate adaptive equipment, like wheelchairs or walkers. Make sure it has the space for mobility devices and seems person centered, and not too fast paced. Consider using personal trainers to help establish an appropriate workout level and schedule. If someone cannot attend a local gym, there are a variety of videos that can be used at home.

When possible, consider accessing community based programs, like local recreational centers and gyms. They usually have a wide variety of activities to meet your needs, and in addition provide socialization and connection with the community at large.

Aerobic Activities

During aerobic activities, the body's large muscles move in a rhythmic manner for a sustained period of time. Aerobic activities help to maintain or improve cardiovascular health. Objectives of aerobic activities include: improving physical fitness and having positive effects on slowness, stiffness, and mood.

Examples of aerobic activities for your loved one:

- Walking
    - With you, a family member, a friend, or your dog
    - On a treadmill
    - On a gentle hike, in a city park
    - Around the shopping mall

- Swimming or water aerobics
    - At your gym or YMCA

- Riding a bike
    - Around the neighborhood or on a stationary bike (also consider tandems and recumbent bikes)

- Dancing
    - At home with you, a family member, or a friend
    - At a local dance hall, club, or ballet center

- Chair aerobics
  - In your living room following along with a video
  - At your local gym or YMCA

Strengthening Activities

Strengthening activities improve muscle strength, walking speed, posture, and overall physical fitness. The objective of improving muscle strength is to facilitate everyday activities such as getting up from a chair, moving from room to room in the home, getting in and out of a car, and making any task easier to manage.

Examples of strengthening activities for your loved one:

- Weights/resistance
  - Free weight activities/exercises
  - Elastic bands activities/exercises
  - Body weight activities/exercises

- Yard work or gardening

- Depending on the hobby, there may be a physical component, for example manual sawing for the individual who enjoys woodworking.

Flexibility Activities

Flexibility or stretching exercises improve mobility, increase range of motion, reduce stiffness, and can help to reduce the risk of injury. Stretching and flexibility activities can improve range of motion, which can affect posture and walking ability, reducing the risk of injury, and making everyday activities easier. Many of these can be tailored to the level your loved one can participate.

Examples of flexibility activities for your loved one:

- Tai chi

- Martial arts like aikido, jujitsu

- Yoga, including chair yoga

Balance Activities

Balance activities can improve posture and stability. Preserving your loved one's ability to maintain balance can help to reduce the likelihood of falling, potentially calm your loved one's fears of falling, and help in performing general daily tasks.

Examples of balance activities for your loved one include:

- Yoga, including chair yoga

- Tai chi

- Water sports like kayaking, paddle boarding

- At-home balance exercises using

  ◦ A Wii

  ◦ A balance ball or balance pillow

Chapter 8

Activities of Daily Living
Tips and Suggestions

Unlike the leisure activities discussed, the activities of daily living covered in this book are necessary activities that are a part of everyday life. The following pages contain tips and suggestions for you to use with your loved one. These are particularly helpful for those at the moderate to total assistance level (see Chapter 3 for descriptions).

Energy Conservation and Rest

The brain requires tremendous energy to heal itself. Energy conservation and rest can be important based on your loved one's unique situation. You have to decide that. As the day is scheduled, make sure to plan periods of rest between activities.

Simplifying daily tasks so your loved one uses less energy can help that person have more energy to do more activities throughout the day. Look at each activity and decide if the way your loved one has always done the activity is the most efficient and uses the least amount of energy. Never underestimate the energy needed for activities requiring a lot of thought or cognition—in addition to the more obvious physical effort required for an activity.

All activities of the day should be planned out to the extent possible—this includes personal care routines, leisure activities, chores, and exercise. They should be spaced throughout the day, with the items that require the most energy being accomplished at the time of day your loved one feels the best.

Do not schedule too many things to do in one day, and be prepared to cancel some plans if your loved one is not feeling well or up to it. It is better to do fewer things over a few days than try to do them all in one day and create exhaustion and pain for three days because of poor pacing.

If your loved one becomes tired during an activity, allow for pause and rest. If your loved one turns a rest period into a nap, be careful not to let the nap go too long during the day, as sleep may become elusive at night. Keeping awake/sleep patterns is important, as are activities.

Bathing

Bathing can be a relaxing, enjoyable experience—or a time of confrontation and anger. If your loved one needs assistance with bathing, use a calm approach. Your loved one's "usual" routine is very important.

Safety and Preparation

- Water temperature should range from 110– 115 degrees Fahrenheit maximum to prevent burning or skin injury.

- Hot water can cause fatigue.

- The floor of the tub needs to be slip proof. Use a rubber mat that doesn't slide, or use permanent nonslip decals.

- Place a nonskid rug on the floor outside the tub to prevent slipping.

- Install grab bars. Always make sure the grab bars are properly and securely installed into the wall studs.

Bathing—Know Your Loved One

- Is your loved one accustomed to a bath or shower?

- Can he/she get into a bath or shower without assistance?

- Can he/she soap the body or wash hair alone?

- Can he/she independently dry with a towel, with simple tricks such as sewing straps onto the towel to make the towel easier to hold?

- If help is needed, who is your loved one the most comfortable with when needing assistance bathing?

- It can be awkward waiting and watching someone perform a task. Instead, the caregiver can provide supervision, but be doing something else. For instance, getting towels out while the loved one is undressing is an effective use of the time and space. Or washing the lower body while the loved one washes upper body deflects this discomfort. This also creates a sense of support versus a feeling of total dependence.

Bathing—Communicating and Motivating

If you have to help a loved one bathe:

- Allow him/her to do what is within that person's control.

- Stay friendly and respectful.

- Try to avoid arguments by offering a combination of visual cues, step-by-step setup, and short verbal cues.

Bathing—Customary Routines and Preferences

- What time of day does your loved one normally bathe?

- How often did your loved one bathe before the injury?

- What is the process that works for you and your loved one when it is time to bathe? Make sure all caregivers know each detail of the process.

  For example, is the water turned on and running prior to your loved one entering the tub? Is a towel placed on a shower chair that your loved one may use so that the chill on his or her bottom is removed when sitting?

- Whatever the process, take it one step at a time, following the person's normal bathing routine. For example, the loved one may prefer that you wash hair first and then body, or soak for 10 minutes before washing.

- When assisting your loved one, have a towel ready to put over the shoulders or on the lap to minimize feelings of exposure.

- Be sure to have your loved one's favorite personal care products for familiar smell and feeling.

<u>Bathing—Planning and Executing</u>

- Have all care items and tools ready prior to starting the bath process.

  ◦ A shower chair if necessary

  ◦ A handheld hose for showering and bathing

- A long-handled sponge or scrubbing brush if self scrubbing is desired

- Sponges with soap inside or a soft soap applicator instead of bar soap (bar soap can easily slip out of your loved one's hand)

- Have a towel and clothing prepared for when the bath is finished.

- A second towel can be placed on the back of a chair to allow your loved one to dry his or her back by rubbing on the towel or you might use a terry cloth robe instead of a towel for drying.

Other Bathroom and Grooming Activities

Encourage loved ones to maintain personal grooming habits. Your loved one may need physical or cognitive assistance or both. If your loved one has participated in occupational therapy, utilize the adaptive and compensatory strategies and tips from rehabilitation for optimum independence. For example, you may need to set up the space so that bathing items are easy to reach, adjust shower seating, or use a handheld shower, a checklist for the steps of the task, or teamwork for the hardest parts of the task.

It can sometimes be easier to "do things" for the loved one to save time and mess. In the long run, this serves to make your loved one more dependent.

- Allow plenty of time for routines. If having your loved one do everything independently takes more time than available, select the two to four tasks that are most important. Keep in mind the big picture. Your loved one may value being outdoors, volunteering, or exercising more. If time is a factor, save time in personal care routines, and spend time on the activities that bring your loved one the most satisfaction.

- Having someone brush your loved one's teeth is not always a comfortable feeling. Always allow him or her to do what is possible. Adaptive grips might help for holding onto the toothbrush. Electric brushes can compensate for fine motor deficits and often include a timer indicating how long to brush.

- Maintaining oral hygiene is very important for those who can no longer do it themselves or do thoroughly. Poor hygiene can lead to additional health problems including gum disease, mouth sores, and infections.

Encourage loved ones to keep up with personal grooming such as shaving, makeup application, and hair care. Provide physical assistance as needed. Large grip items may help with fine motor challenges.

- Use an electric razor for safety.

- Give positive feedback, and avoid pointing out small mistakes.

- If your loved one had been accustomed to wearing makeup, there is no reason for this to stop. If your loved one shows interest or a desire to wear makeup, encourage the familiar routine and offer assistance to apply it if needed. Explore built-up grips for brushes and combs. Consider stabilizing the elbow on the counter or sink to provide more control in the hand.

Hair

- Try to maintain hairstyle and care as your loved one did. However, if independence is more important, consider a style that allows independence. A shorter cut sometimes requires less work and finesse to maintain.

Toileting or Using the Bathroom

- Learn your loved one's individual habits and routines for using the toilet. This might not be something that you knew before and is part of the changing roles.

- Toilet routinely on rising, about 30 to 40 minutes after meals and at bedtime, at minimum.

- If your loved one is having trouble communicating, please watch for agitation, pulling at the clothes, or restlessness. This may be an indication of a need to go to the bathroom.

- Assist with clothing as needed, and be positive and pleasant while assisting.

- Provide verbal cues and instructions as needed. Be guiding, but not controlling.

- If your loved one has fine motor deficits or hemiplegia, consider clothing with minimal fasteners, such as elastic-waist pants or stretch pants that can be pulled up/down.

- Make sure other care providers are aware of toileting schedules on outings.

- Know the public toilet access prior to going somewhere. Not all public bathrooms are user friendly, despite being "accessible."

Clothing

Clothing—Know Your Loved One

- Your loved one may return to the same style of clothes worn before the injury.

- If personal care is a challenge, clothes need to be comfortable and easy to remove, especially to go to bathroom.

- Choose clothes that are loose fitting and have elastic waistbands.

- If possible, choose clothing that opens in the front, not the back. This prevents your loved one from having to reach behind the body and allows the feeling of independence from dressing one's self.

- For those individuals with motor deficits, when purchasing new clothes, look for clothing with large, flat buttons; Velcro closures; or zippers.

- To assist your loved one with zipping pants or a jacket, attach a zipper pull or leather loop on the end of the zipper.

- If bending and tying shoes is problematic, consider slip-on shoes. Non-tie shoes are very popular now.

Clothing—Routines and Preferences

- If your loved one has trouble paying attention and making choices, you may have to limit the choice of clothing, and leave only two outfit options in the room at a time.

- If your loved one wants to wear the same thing every day, and if you can afford it, buy three or four sets of the same clothing.

Clothing—Planning and Executing

- Clothes should be laid out according to what goes on first.

- Avoid clothes that are most difficult for your loved one—such as panty hose, knee-high nylons, tight socks, or high heels.

- Make sure that items are not inside out and that buttons, zips, and fasteners are all undone before handing the clothes to your loved one.

Dressing

Dressing—Know Your Loved One

Your loved one may just need verbal cues and instructions on dressing. Please remember to allow independent dressing as much as possible to foster an ongoing sense of dignity and independence. As the primary caregiver, you will have to be the judge as to when all caregivers need to begin assisting your loved one with dressing.

Dressing—Communicating and Motivating

- Use short, simple sentences, and provide instruction as needed.

- If your loved one is confused, give instructions in very short steps, such as, "Now put your arm through the sleeve." It may help to use actions to demonstrate these instructions.

- Remember to inquire about going to the toilet before getting dressed.

- Avoid "hovering" while your loved one is dressing. You need to be available as needed during the process, but you can do something like making the bed or straightening up so your loved one does not feel so slow, incompetent, or that you are waiting on them.

Dressing—Routines and Preferences

- Does your loved one get dressed first thing in the morning—before breakfast or after breakfast?

- Does your loved one change into pajamas right before bed or after dinner?

- Try to maintain your loved one's preferred routine for as long as possible.

- Little things matter. For example, your loved one may like to put on all underwear before putting on anything else.

Dressing—Planning and Executing

- Think about privacy. Make sure that blinds or curtains are closed and that no one will walk in and disturb your loved one while dressing.

If mistakes are made—for example, by putting something on the wrong way—be tactful, or find a way for both of you to laugh about it.

*Note: Wearing several layers of thin clothing rather than one thick layer can be helpful. With layers, your loved one will be able to remove a layer if too warm.

Remember that your loved one may not be able to tell you if he or she gets too hot or cold, so keep an eye out for signs of discomfort.

Eating

Eating—Know Your Loved One

- Keep long-standing personal preferences in mind when preparing food. However, be aware that your loved one may suddenly develop new food preferences or reject foods that were enjoyed in the past.

- Can your loved one eat independently?

- Does your loved one have a visual impairment that may affect the ability to see a meal or drink? Due to normal changes in our eyesight as we age, eating and dining may offer additional challenges.

Eating—Communicating and Motivating

- Use short, simple sentences.

- Provide verbal cues and instructions as needed.

- Give your loved one your full attention.

- Be guiding, but not controlling.

Eating—Routines and Preferences

- Factor into the overall schedule of the day that it may take an hour or longer to finish each meal or snack.

- Keep mealtimes as simple and familiar as prior to the TBI.

- If eating out was common, consider restaurant accessibility. Try to avoid rush hour if extra time is needed. Make sure to get seating that fits a wheelchair or that optimizes independence.

*Note: Your loved one's sense of taste may change. Food that was eaten for years may no longer be enjoyable. Make note of any changes in your loved one's food preferences on the Personal History Form.

Eating—Planning and Executing

This simple, everyday activity requires maneuvering objects, a skill that many of us may take for granted. You and your loved one will need to develop techniques that work for your loved one.

- It is completely appropriate to ask your loved one if assistance is desired.

- Offer to dish the food onto your loved one's plate, if needed.

- When cutting food, make sure the pieces are small enough for your loved one to chew and swallow easily.

If there are visual deficits, create clear visual distinctions between the table, dishes, and food.

- Use solid colors with no distracting patterns.

- When pouring a light-colored drink, such as milk, use a dark glass.

- When pouring a dark-colored drink, such as cola, use a white glass.

- Avoid clear glasses. They can disappear from view.

- Use white dishes when eating dark-colored food, and use dark dishes when eating light-colored food.

- To make dishes easier to find on the table, use a tablecloth or placemats that are the opposite color of the dishes.

  *Note: Fiesta ware colors (yellow/tangerine) contrast with most foods so they can be easily seen and will enhance visual perception.

- Use adaptive utensils if needed.

- Use a long straw with a no-spill cup or use a plastic mug with a large handle.

Other Meal Considerations

- If temperature discrepancy is limited, test the temperature of foods and beverages before serving.

- Make meals an enjoyable social event, so everyone looks forward to the experience.

- Clean up spills immediately.

- If your loved one wants to assist in making a meal, accommodate.

Meal Preparation Tips
for Someone with Mild TBI

- Labeling cabinets can improve independence for locating items.

- Use simple, step-by-step written or verbal instructions.

- Consider writing out steps and checking off tasks as completed.

- Use proper equipment and modifications for cutting food. There are a variety of adaptive cooking tools from specialized cutting boards for one-handed individuals, built-up utensils, electric can openers, timers for memory problems, to mats for stabilizing equipment.

- Provide supervision and/or assistance as needed for safety.

- When using a stove top, use the back burners, and turn the handles inward toward the back of the stove to avoid any potential grabbing of the pots or pans.

- If you are not there to supervise because you have to go to work, consider structuring and setting up the parts of the task such that your loved one can safely and independently complete them.

- If your loved one is able to manage basic food preparation, but stove top cooking and/or cutting is problematic, put individual meals in a microwaveable container with a label for cook time—or plan cold meals such as sandwiches.

Chapter 9

Home Preparation

Whether you live in a house, an apartment, or an independent living facility, you and your loved one need to feel comfortable, capable, and safe. This is a key foundational piece in preparing to have your loved one engage in any activity. The following are general tips that caregivers and family members can use to prepare the home to accommodate your loved one's needs.

General Organization and Environment

When organizing your loved one's environment, be sure to do it <u>with</u> that person. What works for you might not work for your loved one. Home modifications will depend on the residual challenges faced by your loved one, whether physical or cognitive, and the extent your loved one can independently participate in home activities.

If organization, memory, and attention are an issue, consider:

- Minimizing clutter—putting things back in respective places after use.

- Labeling drawers for items like underwear, pants, socks, etc. (in the kitchen, labeling cabinets).

- Having a set work area for your loved one.

- Putting out reminders—"turn out light, turn off stove, turn on alarm"— as needed.

- Organizing like objects in the same area whenever possible, so that they are easily located.

- If mobility is challenging—providing a walker, cane, or wheelchair.

- Keeping walkways as clear as possible and removing objects frequently left on the floor, such as shoes, bags, and boxes.

They should be placed in their designated areas of the home; if left out, they can be a tripping hazard.

- Using extension cords sparingly, and always securing them out of the places where people walk. Bundle all the cords, and secure them to the wall instead of the floor.

- Removing and avoiding clutter on desks, tables, and countertops, and in cabinets and closets. This makes it easier to locate and reach specific items.

- Avoiding using throw rugs. Although they can make for good identifying markers or nice decorative pieces, they can also be a tripping hazard when your loved one is moving from room to room. If you must use them, opt for slide-resistant rugs that can be taped or tacked down.

- Installing handrails where possible for easier independent movement from one room to the next.

- Identifying and addressing flooring issues. Check every floor, walkway, threshold, and entry. Remove or fix loose floorboards, uneven tiles, loose nails, or carpeting that has bunched up over time.

Furniture

- Make sure there is enough room to move around. If possible, place furniture pieces 5½ feet from each other, so your loved one can move comfortably around the room, especially if in a wheelchair.

- Where possible, arrange your furniture so outlets are easily accessible for lamps and other electrical items without the need for extension cords.

- Use chairs with straight backs, armrests, and firm seats. Where possible, add firm cushions to existing pieces to add height. This will make it easier for your loved one to sit down and get up.

Lighting

Depending on your loved one's vision, the severity of the brain injury, or individual preferences, you may find it necessary to modify existing lighting in the home. These changes could be key in your loved one's safety and ability to perform tasks independently.

- Fluorescent lighting can contribute to an increase in glare. Try different types of lightbulbs to see which is most comfortable for your loved one.

- Keep all rooms evenly lit and the lighting level consistent throughout the home, so shadows and dangerous bright spots are eliminated.

- Make sure light switches, pull cords, and lamps are easily accessible for your loved one particularly if he or she is in a wheelchair.

- If possible, purchase touch lamps or those that can be turned on or off by sound.

- Be certain that all stairwells are well lit and have handrails.

- Depending on the individual, additional task lighting may be necessary in certain areas of the home.

- Additional lighting for closets and smaller areas may be helpful. Battery-operated push lights are a good option.

Glare

Glare can be caused by sunlight or light from a lamp. When light hits a shiny surface, such as a magazine page or even a wall painted with high-gloss paint, the resulting glare can make it difficult for someone with low vision to see.

Sunglasses can be beneficial, both indoors and outside, for someone who is light sensitive.

Offer your loved one an opportunity to try different lens colors to see which works best.

- Sunlight can fill the room with light without producing glare. Adjust sunlight coming through windows by using mini blinds and altering their position throughout the day. If mini blinds are not available, use sheer curtains to diffuse the light.

- Be aware when placing mirrors in a room. Mirrors placed across from larger windows can significantly increase the amount of light in a room. This could be beneficial for someone who prefers the additional light.

- Cover bare lightbulbs with shades.

- Position chairs and tables so that when your loved one is sitting on a chair or at a table, he or she is not having to look directly at the light coming from a window.

- Cover or remove shiny/reflective surfaces such as floors and tabletops.

Color Contrasts

Using contrast is a good strategy if your loved one has a visual impairment due to a TBI or another cause. The more contrast, the easier it is to find and use objects or activity items around the house.

- Put light-colored objects against a dark background.

- Avoid upholstery with patterns for seated activities. Stripes, plaids, and checks can be visually confusing.

- Opt for solid-colored tables and countertops in a neutral tone. Countertops with busy patterns can make it difficult to locate items and can be more difficult to keep clean.

- In a room with mostly dark tones, place light-colored pillows or chairs in strategic places to help your loved one find things and get around easily.

- Put contrasting stripes on the edges of stairs to make each stair visible and to prevent the stairs from disappearing from view.

Chapter 10

Review

The motor and nonmotor effects of TBI, and their severity, vary with each individual. Memory problems, confusion, attention deficit, poor judgment, loss of balance, diminished vision, mood swings, and depression are just some of the challenges of living with a brain injury. Learning to live with and coming to accept the changes can be difficult, not only for the person who has a TBI, but for family and friends as well. As your loved one's primary caregiver, you are in a unique position to understand and see that your loved one's needs are being met. By taking advantage of offers of assistance from family members, friends, and others who are in a position to carry some of the responsibilities of caregiver, the work of caring for your loved one at home can be made a bit easier. One of the keys to making it all work is ensuring that all caregivers are working from the same page. Reading this book is a good first step in reaching that goal.

There are many things to consider and do when caring for a loved one at home. The home must be a safe place for your loved one. We offer many suggestions for preparing your home so that it is a safe environment, but ultimately the decisions on best preparations and changes needed for your loved one are up to you. We offer guidance for communicating with your loved one, when communication is made more difficult by the effects of a TBI.

We encourage you to make every effort to identify, plan, and incorporate activities for your loved one into each day. Meaningful, person-appropriate activities can improve the quality of life for both you and your loved one. There are so many benefits to an Activity Program for your loved one, and you have the opportunity to enjoy them all. If you keep in mind our Four Pillars of Activities as you consider the many activity possibilities, you will be able to choose and implement the activities that are best suited for your loved one.

Following, again, are the Four Pillars of Activities:

First Pillar of Activities: Know your Loved One—Information Gathering and Assessment

- Have a Personal History Form completed.

- Know them—who they are, who they were, and what their functional abilities are today.

- Make sure all caregivers know this information as well.

Second Pillar of Activities: Communicating and Motivating for Success

- Communication is key. Each caregiver must know how to effectively communicate with your loved one and be consistent with techniques.

Third Pillar of Activities: Customary Routines and Preferences

- As best as possible, maintain a routine and daily plan based on your loved one's needs and preferences.

Fourth Pillar of Activities: Planning and Executing Activities

- Based on all of the information you have gathered about your loved one, you have the opportunity to offer engaging activities that are appropriate and meet your loved one's personal preferences.

About the Authors

Scott Silknitter

Scott Silknitter is the founder of R.O.S. Therapy Systems. He designed and created the R.O.S. Play Therapy™ System, the *How Much Do You Know About* Series of themed activity books and the R.O.S. *BIG Book*. Starting with a simple backyard project to help Mom and Dad, Scott has dedicated his life to improving the quality of life for all seniors through meaningful education, entertainment and activities.

Lisa Gonzalez, MS, OT/L, CCM, CBIS

Lisa is an occupational therapist and certified case manager. She is also a certified brain injury specialist through ACBIS. She has more than 20 years of experience as a clinical OT servicing a variety of areas including home health, skilled nursing, and acute care. In addition, she was an OTA instructor for Durham Technical Community College for 5 years and remains on the advisory board for that program. For the majority of her career, Lisa served as an OT and activity program coordinator in a residential community re-entry program for individuals with TBI. She currently works as a case manager for NeuroCommunity Care—providing community-based support services for individuals with TBI. Lisa and her team proudly serve wounded veterans and their families nationwide. With her current team, Lisa helps injured veterans and their families dealing with Traumatic Brain Injury access community-based resources and services designed to improve their quality of life and foster stabilization.

M. Heather McKay, MS, OT/L

Heather is an award-winning occupational therapist and dementia care specialist, consultant, and international trainer/speaker providing training for professional and family caregivers, services to individuals with aging issues, and consultation with facilities on topics related to dementia and Alzheimer's care. Heather collaborated with national and local veteran groups to produce the acclaimed film series *Dementia Care for America's Heroes,* featuring family caregivers in the Long Island State Veterans Home. Heather proudly works with veterans and their caregivers in Veterans' Homes nationwide.

References

1. *The Handbook of Theories on Aging* (Bengtson, *et al.*, 2009)
2. *Activity Keeps Me Going*, Volume A, (Peckham, *et al.*, 2011)
3. *Essentials for the Activity Professional in Long-Term Care* (Lanza, 1997)
4. *Abnormal Psychology*, Butcher
5. www.dhspecialservices.com
6. National Certification Council for Dementia Practitioners www.NCCDP.org
7. *Managing Difficult Dementia Behaviors: An A-B-C Approach* by Carrie Steckl
8. Iowa Geriatric Education Center website, Marianne Smith, PhD, ARNP, BC Assistant Professor University of Iowa College of Nursing
9. *Excerpts taken from "Behavior...Whose Problem is it?" Hommel, 2012
10. Merriam-Webster's dictionary
11. *The Latent Kin Matrix* (Riley, 1983)
12. *Care Planning Cookbook* (Nolta, *et al.*, 2007)
13. *Long-Term Care* (Blasko, *et al.*, 2011)
14. *Success Oriented Programs for the Dementia Client* (Worsley, *et al.*, 2005)
15. Heerema, Esther. "Eight Reasons Why Meaningful Activities Are Important for People with Dementia." www.about.com
16. Activities 101 for the Family Caregiver (Appler-Worsley, Bradshaw, Silknitter)
17. American Foundation for the Blind
18. www.aging.com
19. www.WebMD.com
20. www.caregiver.org

21. AOTA Tip Sheet Adults with Traumatic Brain Injury http://www.aota.org/about-occupational-therapy/patients-clients/disabilityandrehabilitation/tbi.aspx

22. Armstrong, Lauren. (2009). Out of Synch: The effects of Traumatic Brain Injury (TBI) and the battle to recover. *FRA Today* July: 18-24.

23. Snow, T. (2010). *Enhancing understanding of dementia and building skills for better care and outcomes.* Retrieved Nov. 1, 2012, from http://www.slideshare.net/HISCSonoma/teepa-snow-dementia-building-skill-handout

24. McKay, H., Mangrum Hanzaker, M. (2013). Dementia care communication: A toolbox for professionals and families. *OT Practice,* February 18(3): CE 1-8.

25. Centers for Disease Control and Prevention. Traumatic injury in the United States: Fact Sheet. http://www.cdc.gov/traumaticbraininjury/get_the_facts.html

26. Brainline.org. Facts about Traumatic brain injury. http://www.brainline.org/content/2008/07/facts-about-traumatic-brain-injury.html?gclid=CKCbyMXn6cUCFcURHwodUA4AIA

27. Ranchos Los Amigos- Revised Levels of Cognitive Functioning. http://www.coma.ulg.ac.be/images/levels_cogfunc.pdf

28. Wright, J. (2000). The Functional Assessment Measure. *The Center for Outcome Measurement in Brain Injury.*http://www.tbims.org/combi/FAM (accessed May 30, 2015).*

Family Members and Caregivers
that have read this book:

_____

_____

_____

_____

_____

_____

_____

_____

_____

_____

_____

_____

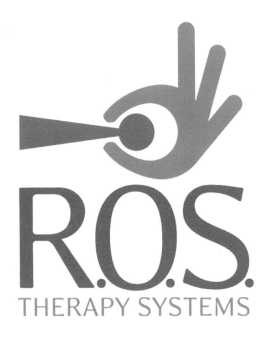

For additional assistance, please contact us at:
www.ROSTherapySystems.com
888-352-9788